The Transitioning Hair Care Manual

A Step By Step Guide To Transition From Relaxed Hair To Natural Hair

AUTHOR BREANNA RUTTER

TABLE OF CONTENTS

INTRODUCTION TO THE TRANSITIONING HAIR CARE MANUAL

"The Transitioning Hair Care Manual is a pocket guide that will help you to successfully transition from relaxed hair to natural hair. You may have chosen to transition with your hair for a variety of reasons; health reasons, a change in appearance, or to just experience your natural hair. Transitioning from relaxed hair to natural hair is a process that involves slowly trimming off your relaxed ends over a period of time until you have 100% natural hair. Understanding how to take care of Transitioning Hair can be quite challenging especially if you do not know where to start or you don't know how to care for your hair to keep it thriving and growing.

This manual breaks down transitioning in easy simple steps with incredibly easy techniques you can implement requiring little to no hair skills. Your transitioning hair care regimen will involve a combination of hair care practices from a natural hair regimen and a relaxed hair regimen since you will or already have both natural hair and relaxed hair!

Working with transitioning hair can be very daunting considering the fact that you have to manage two different textures of hair but as you learn their different needs, taking care of both textures of hair will become second nature, I promise! This manual will point you in the right direction as far as products go but you will soon realize that hair care techniques far exceeds the actual hair products themselves!

Please enjoy this informative read and have fun experiencing the different stages of your hair while transitioning." -Sincerely Breanna

1 HAIR CARE TOOLS

It should be of no surprise that the tools you use to take care of your transitioning hair are extremely important in regards to maintaining healthy hair! There are a wide variety of hair care tools available on the market so don't allow yourself to become overwhelmed by their visual appeal. The most important thing to keep in mind when acquiring your hair care tools, is that they are constructed in a manner that does not compromise the health of your hair. New tools will always rise and fall and even if some actually gain popularity, there is no need to sway from your tools of choice if they meets your needs.

The only hair tool that is necessary for detangling and maintaining groomed transitioning hair is a seamless wide tooth detangling comb! This has always been the #1 secret to great hair no matter how fine, thick, course, silky, curly, straight, or wavy your is, you will always need a wide tooth comb for your detangling & grooming needs! This tool will prevent a great deal of damage & split ends, trust me!

What's also just as important as a seamless wide tooth detangling comb, are a pair of hair cutting shears. The beauty about transitioning hair is that you don't have to cut off all of your hair at once since you are preserving length while transitioning into fully natural hair. To keep transitioning hair in tip top condition though, you have to occasionally trim damaged/splitting ends when necessary and trim off some length of relaxed hair when you are ready. Also since the oldest part of your hair are the ends, it's a normal that overtime, you will experience splitting or slightly damaged ends even if you have very healthy hair!

I will provide a list of safe and harsh hair care tools for you & in a later section, elaborate more on trimming your ends!

SAFE HAIR CARE TOOLS	HARSH HAIR CARE TOOLS
Seamless Wide Tooth Comb	Combs with Seams In-between the Teeth
Soft Boar Bristle Hair Brush	Plastic Bristle Hair Brush
Hair Cutting Shears (only to be used on hair)	Safety Scissors (Household Scissors)
Silk Hair Accessories	Cotton/Wool Hair Accessories
Ouchless/Seamless Hair Bands	Metal Bind/Plastic Bind On Hair Bands
Paddle Brush	Metal Wig Brush
Heat Styling Up To 350°	Heat Styling Over 350°
Blow Drying on Low-Medium Heat	Blow Drying on High Heat

2 DETANGLE

Properly detangling transitioning hair is your first line of defense when protecting yourself from breakage and damage. Use extreme gentleness when detangling your hair because the line of demarcation (refer to definition guide) in your hair is the weakest point of your hair, your relaxed hair is the 2nd weakest, and your new growth hair (natural hair) is the strongest hair you have. When freeing tangles, you must detangle your hair with a wide tooth comb! Sometimes just raking your fingers gently through your hair is enough for loose curly hair types but in most cases, a wide tooth comb is preferred. Also when detangling your hair, doing so as infrequent as possible limits your chances of hair damage because the more you handle your hair, the easier hair damage can occur. It is best to only detangle your hair prior to shampoo washing or before a hair treatment, or before styling to keep detangling at a minimum. Also, wearing styles that last until your next shampoo or conditioner wash limits detangling even more.

Detangling your transitioning hair will differ depending on how tight of a curl your natural hair has. Straight to wavy new growth can be detangled while dry from tip to root. If you have curly to coily new growth hair, you should detangle your relaxed hair dry first and then your new growth while wet. The reason why relaxed hair should be detangled dry & your roots wet, is because relaxed hair has a tendency to tangle/mat when wet. Hair with a looser curl can follow a detangle process just like curly to coily hair, but this is not needed. In most cases, loose curly hair can be detangled dry from tip to root with ease!

I will walk you step by step through how to detangle your hair properly no matter the texture or curl pattern of your transitioning hair!

8

Transitioning Hair Detangle Regimen

Step #1 Dry detangle relaxed ends in manageable sections (6-8 sections) from the tips to the line of demarcation, with a seamless wide tooth comb

(Loose Curly Hair) Continue to thoroughly detangle sections past the line of demarcation while hair is dry

Step #2 (Curly to Coily Hair) Generously apply your rinse conditioner to your natural hair (roots) and wait a couple of minutes until your hair has softened

Step #3 Per section, gently detangle your natural hair by starting at the line of demarcation and following through to the ends. Continue each detangling stroke higher up your new growth until you reach your scalp. The last detangling stroke is when you can successfully comb once with ease through your section of hair!

Step #4 Loosely braid or twist each section and rinse out all traces of conditioner with warm water

Step #5 Final rinse with the coolest water you can stand to close your cuticles for smooth frizz free hair

Step #6 Pat towel dry, unravel your sections, and proceed to follow up with styling or follow up with your hair treatment of choice!

3 SHAMPOO

When shampooing transitioning hair, understand that a little shampoo goes a long way! In fact, black hair does not have to be shampooed as often as other hair types and because of this, there is the added pressure of finding the perfect shampoo that will not strip your hair of vital moisture. Commercial shampoos are usually filled with very stripping cleansing agents that often leave your hair dryer after shampooing. Using a mild shampoo is all around better for preserving the health of your hair because of its mild cleansing power. Additionally, every time you shampoo wash your hair, it is highly advisable that you perform a Deep Condition Treatment but if your shampoo does not cause a squeaky clean finish, skipping a Deep Conditioning Treatment is just fine!

A good guide for knowing how often to shampoo wash transitioning hair is at least once a week or once every two weeks. This will vary depending on the frequency of your hair product usage and the condition of your scalp and hair. In any case, even if you work out, do not shampoo your hair more than once a week. Instead, conditioner wash in the middle of the week and shampoo wash at the end of the week. You can of course only shampoo wash according to your unique needs (which would be best) by paying attention to notice buildup of hair products, dandruff, odor, or an itchy scalp. Any or all of the above are good indicators that it would be a good time to shampoo wash your hair.

I will walk you step by step through how to shampoo wash your hair and if you are in need of a quality shampoo, I highly suggest HowToBlackHair.com referred hair care products specifically formulated for maintaining healthy hair.

Transitioning Hair Shampoo Regimen

Step #1 Follow the Transitioning Hair Detangle Regimen but skip Steps 5 & 6

Step #2 Apply shampoo directly to the scalp and message with finger pads to form a lather

Step #3 Unravel a section and use lather to cleanse the ends then lightly re-braid or re-twist your section. Repeat this step on all sections, one at a time

Step #4 Rinse all traces of shampoo from hair with warm water

Step #5 Final rinse with the coolest water you can stand to close your cuticles for smooth frizz free hair

Step #6 Pat towel dry, unravel your sections, and proceed to follow up with styling or your hair treatment of choice!

4 DEEP CONDITION

Transitioning hair requires deep condition treatments to keep it healthy, especially when it comes to preserving the health of your relaxed ends! Relaxed hair is a weakened state of your hair because it takes the use of a chemical relaxer to damage your hair, to a degree, for desired straightness. This treatment compromises many layers of the hair shaft and in doing so, this leaves your hair lacking in protein and moisture. That's why a shaft penetrating conditioner is a necessary treatment you must incorporate into your regimen, if you want to successfully transition with your hair.

Using a deep conditioner product will not be done frequently but, it is vital for balancing much needed moisture into your hair. You will usually notice that during the hotter & drier times of year, more deep conditioning is required to quench dry hair!

A good guide for knowing how often to deep condition your hair is at least every week or every two weeks. Deep conditioning your hair will vary sometimes depending on how tight your curl pattern is, your hair care styling habits, & usage of other hair products as well. Also, while deep conditioning your hair, remember to avoid adding product to your scalp as this causes buildup!

Next, I will walk you step by step through how to deep condition your hair properly from start to finish! If you are in need of a quality deep conditioner for your transitioning hair, I highly suggest HowToBlackHair.com referred hair care products specifically formulated for maintaining healthy hair.

Transitioning Hair Deep Condition Regimen

Step #1 Dry detangle relaxed ends in manageable sections (6-8 sections) from the tips to the line of demarcation, with a seamless wide tooth comb

(Loose Curly Hair) Continue to thoroughly detangle sections past the line of demarcation while hair is dry

Step #2 (Curly to Coily Hair) Generously apply your deep conditioner to your natural hair and wait a couple of minutes until your hair has softened

Step #3 Per section, gently detangle your natural hair by starting at the line of demarcation and following through to the ends. Continue each detangling stroke higher up your new growth until you reach your scalp. The last detangling stroke is when you can successfully comb once with ease through your section of hair!

Step #4 Saturate the ends with product & loosely braid or twist each section. Deep condition as suggested by the product or cover your hair with a shower cap and process for 30 minutes max

Step #5 Thoroughly rinse hair with warm water & final rinse with cool water to close your cuticles for smooth frizz free hair

Step #6 Pat towel dry, unravel your sections, and proceed to follow up with your styling of choice!

5 PROTEIN TREATMENT

Protein treatments serve as a corrective treatment for transitioning hair since relaxed hair has a tendency to lack strength. To restore elasticity on the other hand, deep conditioners specifically serve that purpose for your hair. Similar to a deep conditioner, you need a protein treatment that has the ability to penetrate your hair shaft to make it stronger from the inside out. Transitioning hair by nature, desperately needs a protein treatment to prevent relaxed hair from breaking! Natural hair on the other hand, is stronger because it has not been stripped of its protein so applying protein that is not needed to natural hair, will make it stiff or crunchy to touch! Protein treatments are still to be taken with caution on relaxed ends because hair that has too much protein can cause breakage because its elasticity has been compromised.

A good guide for knowing how often to do a protein treatment on the relaxed part of your transitioning hair will depend on the state of your relaxed ends since this is the only hair that requires a steady supply of protein. It is recommended to protein treat relaxed hair every two weeks while transitioning. If limp, lifeless, or very stretchy describes the state of your hair, you are in serious need of a protein treatment! The easiest way to tell if a protein treatment is needed is most noticeable directly after shampoo washing your hair.

I will walk you step by step through how to protein treat your hair properly and if you are in need of a quality protein conditioning treatment for your transitioning hair, I highly suggest HowToBlackHair.com referred hair care products specifically formulated for maintaining healthy hair.

Transitioning Hair Protein Treatment Regimen

Step #1 Follow the Transitioning Hair Detangle Regimen but allow hair to air dry while in sections

Step #2 Per section, saturate the ends with your protein treatment & loosely re-braid or re-twist each section. Protein treat as suggested by the product or cover your hair with a shower cap to process for 30 minutes max

*For Intense Results: cover hair with a shower cap and protein treat for a max time of 30 minutes under a hooded dryer. This is necessary in the case of treating extremely damaged relaxed hair!

Step #3 Thoroughly rinse out all traces of the protein treatment from your hair with warm water & final rinse with the coolest water you can stand to close your cuticles for smooth frizz free hair

Step #4 Pat towel dry, unravel your sections, and proceed to follow up with your styling of choice!

6 CONDITIONER WASH

No matter if your hair is color treated, heat trained, natural, or chemically relaxed, black hair always needs a steady supply of moisture. Healthy transitioning hair that is kept moisturized, prevents it from becoming dry which leads to splitting breaking ends! The key to any successful hair care regimen believe it or not, is an incorporation of co-washing. Co-wash means to wash your hair with conditioner alone and this is a great way to re-moisturize your hair when you are noticing that your hair is becoming dry but is not in need of a shampoo wash. Preferably, use an inexpensive water based conditioning product to serve as your co-wash conditioner and to also aid you with detangling. Rinse Conditioners/Co Wash Conditioners are usually used frequently and in large quantities so having an adequate supply of this conditioner is important when helping you maintain the health of your hair.

A good guide for knowing how often to conditioner wash transitioning hair is at least twice a week or weekly. The frequency of your co-washes will depend on how well your hair can retain moisture as well as how physically active your lifestyle is. Tighter curl patterns (like Type 4 Hair) often need more moisturizing care than a looser curl pattern (like Type 3 Hair). You can of course only co-wash according to your unique needs (which would be best) by paying attention to notice if your hair is feeling drier than normal. Co-washing is also a way to cleanse your hair when needed, but co-washing cannot replace your shampoo wash!

I will walk you step by step through how to co-wash your hair and if you are in need of a quality conditioner for your transitioning hair, I highly suggest HowToBlackHair.com referred hair care products specifically formulated for maintaining healthy hair.

Transitioning Hair Conditioner Wash Regimen

Step #1 Dry detangle relaxed ends in manageable sections (6-8 sections) from the tips to the line of demarcation, with a seamless wide tooth comb

(Loose Curly Hair) Continue to thoroughly detangle sections past the line of demarcation while hair is dry

Step #2 (Curly to Coily Hair) Generously apply your rinse conditioner to your natural hair (roots) and wait a couple of minutes until your hair has softened

Step #3 Per section, gently detangle your natural hair by starting at the line of demarcation and following through to the ends. Continue each detangling stroke higher up your new growth until you reach your scalp. The last detangling stroke is when you can successfully comb once with ease through your section of hair!

Step #4 Loosely braid or twist each section and rinse out all traces of conditioner with warm water

Step #5 Final rinse with the coolest water you can stand to close your cuticles for smooth frizz free hair

Step #6 Pat towel dry, unravel your sections, and proceed to follow up with styling or follow up with your hair treatment of choice!

7 LEAVE IN MOISTURIZER

For transitioning hair, your leave in moisturizer will serve alone as the purpose for adding moisture into your hair. It has been suggested according to the detangle regimen to detangle with a rinse conditioner/co-wash conditioner but if you want to detangle with a leave in moisturizer instead, that's an option as well. The reason why detangling with a leave in moisturizer was not suggested for the detangle regimen is because leave in moisturizers are designed to moisturize your hair internally while a rinse conditioner is designed to just attract water to the outer surface of your hair, which aids you best when detangling.

A good guide for knowing how often to apply a leave in moisturizer to your hair is bi-weekly or weekly. The frequency of applying a leave in moisturizer to your hair will vary depending on how tight your curl pattern is and how well your hair can retain moisture. Tighter curl patterns (like Type 4 Hair) often need more moisturizing attention than a looser curl pattern (like Type 3 Hair). With this product, you have to experiment applying it on damp or dry hair to find out when applying it to your hair is best. Many transitioners prefer applying a leave in on damp hair because it feels like the product actually absorbs into the hair rather than sit on top of their strands. Also, if your hair tends to still feel dry, try applying your leave in moisturizer with the LOC method. Refer to the definition guide for more information on the LOC Method!

I will walk you step by step through how to moisturize your hair and if you are in need of a quality leave in moisturizer, I highly suggest HowToBlackHair.com referred hair care products specifically formulated for maintaining healthy hair.

Transitioning Hair Leave In Moisturizer Regimen

Step #1 Follow the Transitioning Hair Detangle Regimen but allow hair to air dry while in sections

Step #2 Coat leave in moisturizer, section by section, on detangled hair

Do not apply product to the scalp as this causes buildup!

Step #3 For increased moisture (if you struggle with dry hair) incorporate the LOC Method with your choice of products

Step #4 Proceed to style working on one section at a time. If you like to style dried hair, allow hair to air dry or blow dry preferably with low heat

8 OIL SEALANT

Your choice of an oil sealant will prevent your moisturizing practices from being a waste of time and effort! Throughout this manual, there has been an extreme emphasis placed on keeping transitioning hair supplied with moisture because healthy transitioning hair is synonymous with moisturized hair. The purpose of using an oil sealant in your hair care regimen, is to slow down the rate of water evaporating from the strands of your hair. To clarify, there is no such thing as a permanent sealant that will keep your hair moisturized forever because a sealant like that will most likely damage your hair, prevent you from effectively using heat, and make chemical treatments like coloring and deep conditioning ineffective. Keep in mind that the heavier or thicker your oil sealant of choice is, the longer your hair can retain moisture and the more greasy your hair will feel.

A good guide for knowing how often to use an oil sealant on transitioning hair is before or after applying your leave in moisturizer. If you adopt the LOC Method, sealing your hair with oil will be done before your creamy leave in moisturizer is applied to your hair. Depending on your hair, you may prefer lighter oils like Coconut oil or heavier oils/butters like Castor oil or Shea Butter. For the majority, tighter curl patterns lean more towards heavier oils/butters and looser curl patterns, lean more towards lighter oils. If your hair has a tendency to have a constant dryness, try thicker consistency (heavier) oils/butters and if you don't have much difficulty maintaining moisturized hair, try thinner consistency (lighter) oils as your oil sealant.

I will walk you step by step through how to oil seal your hair and if you are in need of a quality oil sealant, I highly suggest HowToBlackHair.com referred hair care products specifically formulated for maintaining healthy hair.

Transitioning Hair Oil Sealant Regimen

Step #1 (Without the LOC Method for Manageable Hair)

Lightly coat fingers with your oil/butter or choice and lubricate damp hair in manageable sections at a time

Oil seal preferably AFTER applying your creamy leave in moisturizer or Oil seal on damp product free hair

Focus on the ends of your hair as this needs the most coverage when maintaining moisturized transitioning hair!

Step #2 (With the LOC Method for Constant Dry Hair)

Lightly coat fingers with your oil/butter or choice and lubricate manageable sections at a time RIGHT BEFORE applying your creamy leave in moisturizer

After applying your oil, apply your creamy leave in moisturizer to complete the LOC Method

Step #3 Proceed to style working on one section at a time. If you like to style dried hair, allow hair to air dry or blow dry preferably with low heat

9 HAIR GEL

Hair gel is an optional hair product unlike your other hair care products. The previous hair products mentioned are mandatory for a healthy hair care regimen but products like gel, mousse, or holding sprays are 100% optional when you want to use them for styling. Your choice of hair gel in particular, will depend on your styling needs and how well your hair gel will cooperate with your hair products. For a light hold, watery/loose consistency hair gels can provide a little hold but for keeping edges held smooth and slick without waving or reverting to curls, a stronger hold (thicker consistency) gel would be better. Gels can be used to keep your hair slick and smooth and this product can also be used to define your hair to make your curl pattern pop!

A good guide for knowing how to use gel on transitioning hair will depend on your styling needs. The consistency and hold of your hair gel are not synonymous with being best for certain hair textures or curl patterns. Some gels provide light, medium or strong holds according to their labels. Only apply hair gel to moisturized hair to avoid hard hair and be cautious of gels that contain protein in their ingredients list. It is very easy overloading your hair with protein than it is to over moisturize your hair.

I will walk you step by step through how to use hair gel on your transitioning hair and if you are in need of a quality hair gel, I highly suggest HowToBlackHair.com referred hair care products specifically formulated for maintaining healthy hair.

Transitioning Hair Gel Regimen

Step #1 Lightly coat fingers with your hair gel and lubricate manageable sections at a time then proceed to style!

This step is great for curl sets like; Perm Rod Sets, Straw Sets or Flexirod Sets for example

Step #2 (For Sculpted Edges)

Apply your hair gel to your edges and sculpt with the pads of your fingers or a soft toothbrush (commonly used)

Step #4 (Optional)

Tie down your hair (or edges) with a silk head scarf or a molding strip, for at least 5 minutes, to allow your hair to set while drying

10 HAIR CARE REGIMEN

I have explained the purpose of your hair care products, how often to apply them and more importantly, directions on how to apply them! Your hair care regimen for transitioning hair takes on a blend of both Natural Hair and Relaxed Hair Regimens and with patience and a little skill, you will be able to take great care of your hair while transitioning and beyond. As you may have observed, taking care of transitioning hair has to always be done in sections being that there is a preferred way in detangling relaxed hair verses natural hair. Understanding how to do a variety of simple hair care techniques all contribute to your overall hair care regimen.

So of course it's almost a given that you still do not understand how to implement a regimen that will work for you because from each suggested product regimen, it can make you feel overwhelmed as well as leave you to assume that you have to handle your hair frequently, which is actually the opposite.

Follow along with the suggested weekly hair care regimen that will be explained next and keep in mind that the chart is 100% flexible to your unique hair care needs. One day you may feel the need to tweak certain parts of the hair care regimen so feel free to make changes that are necessary for you.

I will walk you step by step through an awesome hair care regimen that you can use as a guide for taking care of your transitioning hair and in the following sections, we will discuss various hairstyling options as well as how to handle the disappointments many individuals go through when transitioning to natural hair.

Transitioning Hair Care Regimen	
(WEEK 1/DAY 1) *Detangle(mandatory) *Shampoo(mandatory) *Deep Condition (mandatory) *Leave In Moisturizer (mandatory) *Oil Sealant (mandatory) *Hair Gel (optional)	(WEEK 2/DAY 1) *Detangle(mandatory) *Shampoo(mandatory) *Protein Treatment (mandatory) *Leave In Moisturizer (mandatory) *Oil Sealant (mandatory) *Hair Gel (optional)
(WEEK 1/DAY 2)	(WEEK 2/DAY 2)
(WEEK 1/DAY 3)	(WEEK 2/DAY 3)
(WEEK 1/DAY 4) *Conditioner Wash(optional) *Leave In Moisturizer (optional) *Oil Sealant (optional) *Hair Gel (optional)	(WEEK 2/DAY 4) *Conditioner Wash(optional) *Leave In Moisturizer (optional) *Oil Sealant (optional) *Hair Gel (optional)
(WEEK 1/DAY 5)	(WEEK 2/DAY 5)
(WEEK 1/DAY 6)	(WEEK 2/DAY 6)
(WEEK 1/DAY 7) *Conditioner Wash(optional) *Leave In Moisturizer (optional) *Oil Sealant (optional) *Hair Gel (optional)	(WEEK 1/DAY 7) *Conditioner Wash(optional) *Leave In Moisturizer (optional) *Oil Sealant (optional) *Hair Gel (optional)
Continue to repeat this 2 WEEK Cycle Feel free to moisturize more frequently if necessary	

11 HAIRSTYLING OPTIONS

Opposite to what many people think, transitioning hair has a variety of versatile hairstyles that can make transitioning hair look just as beautiful in styles as natural hair. The main reason why many individuals think that transitioning hair does not offer much variety of styling, is because blending two different textures of hair into one look can be quite challenging! Taming your roots down to help blend with the state of your relaxed hair, takes some trial and error as well as patience to achieve the look you truly want. The problem with many natural hairstyles on transitioning hair is that your natural hair usually looks more voluminous while you relaxed ends look straighter and sometimes silkier. There are so many ways to make natural hairstyles on your transitioning hair look flawless and I will teach you how!

Before I begin to teach you how to achieve natural hairstyles on transitioning hair, I will first address wearing weaves and extensions on transitioning hair. For many long term transtitioners, weaves and extensions have been their secret to successfully growing their hair without major setbacks, but added extension and weaving hair can cause drastic breakage! The problem with wearing weave and extensions is that first and foremost, the added weight of additional hair on your strands can dramatically weaken your hair. Fine and/or damaged hair is prone to breakage when adding additional hair onto your real hair. Also, since installs cause you to see your hair infrequently, this can cause an imbalance of moisture & protein which leads right towards breakage! Wearing installs should be left to your judgment when your hair is in a healthy state because it works for some, and causes problems for others.

DEEP WAVES

(No Heat) Take chunky sections of damp moisturized hair & secure wave rollers onto your sections. You can also achieve waves by braiding chunky braids on damp moisturized hair & unravel them when dry.

PERM ROD SET

(No Heat) Take sections of damp moisturized hair a little less wide than your perm rod & rotate the perm rod on your ends first (using gel is optional for curls with hold). After rolling the end of your section in a way that tucks your ends, continue rolling hair against the surface of the rod. Secure the plunger & allow hair to dry overnight as you sleep in a silk scarf or bonnet. Unravel rods in the opposite direction as to not disturb your curls. If desired, separate each curl for bigger hair!

FLEXI ROD SET

(No Heat) Take small to medium sections of damp moisturized hair & rotate the flexi on your ends. After rolling the end of your section in a way that tucks your ends, continue rolling hair against the surface of the flexi. Fold the top of the flexi downward, over your hair, to secure & allow hair to dry overnight. Unravel flexi rods in the opposite direction as to not disturb your curls. If desired, separate each curl for bigger hair!

For more hairstyling options, visit our hair care & styling website at HowToBlackHair.com!

12 HEAT DAMAGE

The fastest way to damage transitioning hair and cause massive breakage is by inflicting heat damage! Heat damaged hair is common with many who transition from relaxed hair to natural hair, because this is the easiest but most damaging way to straighten hair. Keep in mind that the visible hair seen on your head is dead because its cells are no longer alive so hair is like a shell filled with your natural hair color. Your hair can only temporarily hold added proteins and are lost constantly on a small scale. That is why one protein treatment on relaxed hair is not enough, adding protein weekly to hair mimics the strength it naturally had before relaxing your hair.

Heat styling on the other hand changes the structure of your hair when the heat used is intolerable. That's why one individual can take a heat temperature of 350°and another individual cannot go over 300° not because their hair is unhealthy, but because everyone's hair has a different level of heat tolerance. It is not suggested to use heat on transitioning hair, even at safe temperatures, because your relaxed and natural hair has a different level of tolerance. If you must use heat, seldom is best but all in all, styling your hair without heat will work best for you in the long run towards healthy hair.

I will walk you step by step through using heat safely on your transitioning hair, if you must. If you are in need of a quality heat protectant, I highly suggest HowToBlackHair.com referred hair care products specifically formulated for maintaining healthy hair.

ONLY USE HEAT ON HEALTHY TRANSITIONING HAIR!

(BLOW DRYING) Blow dry in manageable sections (6 to 8 sections) preferably on low heat with the tension method (refer to definition guide)

(HOODED DRYER/BONNET DRYER) Use heat to dry your curl sets faster, preferably on low heat until dry

(FLAT IRON/STRAIGHTNER) With dry moisturized hair, lubricate hair with your heat protectant primarily focusing on the ends of your relaxed hair. Preferably start at temperatures 250° to 300° on your flat iron and slowly increase heat setting to no higher than 350° for desired straightness.

Use the Chase Method to limit your passes with your flat iron (refer to the definition guide)

To avoid heat damage, patch test! Take a small amount of hair in an area of your head that is usually not seen through your hairstyles, and start low then increase in heat temperature with your straightener to reach your desired straightness. Allow hair to cool and thoroughly saturate your straightened hair with water and a little bit of shampoo to see if your hair reverts. Allow at least 10 minutes to check your final results. If your natural hair returns back to its curl pattern, heat damage has not occurred!

13 BREAKAGE

Caring for broken transitioning hair has caused many to opt for the Big Chop (discussed in a later section) than deal with the frustration of overcoming hair breakage. Breakage can happen for a variety of reasons with some being natural occurrences and others being completely your fault! Over time, hair naturally becomes courser and drier near the ends, being that it is the oldest part of your hair that has endured the most manipulation over time. The ends of your hair will become more dry and course but that doesn't mean it is damaged. A simple Protein Treatment or Deep Condition can make your ends feel brand new all over again and when this doesn't quite work, its suggested to trim or dust the ends of your hair (discussed in a later section).

Breakage can also occur from Hairstyling or Detangling as manipulation heightens your chances of breakage. Combing your hair is not a bad thing, its actually required in preventing your hair from matting, but manipulation no matter how gentle, wears down on the health of end hairs over time. That's why it so important to handle your hair as infrequent as possible (preferably weekly) and to always use gentleness to achieve what you want. When detangling, do not rip through your hair! If you reach a knot or very resistant pass through your hair, gently comb through the bottom most part of the resistance to stop breakage from occurring. When styling, use little to no heat and gently smooth your hair when necessary as this prevents breakage from happening in the long run as well!

In the next section, we will elaborate on how to trim your ends to maintain healthy transitioning hair.

14 TRIMMING RELAXED ENDS

Transitioning hair has to eventually come to an end and it doesn't have to be done drastically, but ridding of your relaxed ends should be an important goal to achieve with your unique level of comfort. Even though your seamless wide tooth detangling comb is your most important hair tool, your cutting shears are just as important because it brings healthy ends as well as one step closer to 100% natural hair!

As mentioned previously, trimming your relaxed ends does not mean that you have to big chop whatsoever, you just have to gradually trim your ends to your level of comfort. Some transitioners like to trim their hair in line of maintaining their length. For example, say you have been transitioning and you have grown 5 inches of new growth (stretched) with 10 inches of relaxed hair. Some will trim off 5 inches of relaxed hair if they have reached 5 inches of new growth, which keeps you at the length of 10 inches of hair altogether. Then once your natural hair has reached 10 inches (stretched) the rest of their relaxed hair is trimmed off leaving them with 100% natural hair that is 10 inches long. The surprise that comes along with doing this is that your hair will look significantly shorter with 10 inches of natural hair in comparison to 10 inches of relaxed hair because of shrinkage! Natural hair can shrink in length anywhere from 30% to 70% of your actual length and in this case, 10 inches of un-stretched natural hair will look like 3 to 7 inches of hair! For an easier adjustment, trim off about a 1/4 inch of relaxed hair per 1 inch of new growth gain.

I will walk you step by step through how to trim your relaxed ends as well as trim damaged ends!

ONLY USE CUTTING SHEARS EXCLUSIVELY
ON YOUR TRANSITIONING HAIR!

(TRIMMING DAMAGED ENDS)

Step #1 Dust trim detangled relaxed ends while wet in small sections at a time, making sure to do so in a well lit room with mirrors to help.

Step #2 Starting in the back of your head, part a horizontal line of hair at the nape of your neck and use gator clips or duck bill clips to keep the rest of your hair sectioned out of the way. Always dust small sections at a time.

Step #3 Take a small section of detangled hair, twist to the ends, and trim about an 1/8 inch of hair to dust for maintenance. Your dusted hair ends should look like little flecks of hair. For a trim that requires more than an 1/8 of length lost, consult with a professional to aid you so that you don't accidently give yourself an uneven trim.

(TRIMMING RELAXED HAIR)

Step #1 Fist decide how much length of relaxed hair you are willing to lose because losing a lot of relaxed hair at once can be difficult to deal with.

Step #2 Follow Step 2 from above but trim off your desired length. If you feel as though you need assistance, consult with a professional to aid you so that you don't accidently give yourself an uneven trim or haircut!

15 BIG CHOP

While transitioning with your hair, it is only natural that Big Chopping your hair comes across your mind from time to time. Some transitioners are afraid to Big Chop and avoid doing so at all costs, that is perfectly fine. What is not okay is refusing to at least trim splitting damaged ends for the sake of saving length. Avoiding trims or dusting for maintaining healthy ends was heavily discussed in both previous books, The Natural Hair Bible and The Relaxed Hair Bible. When you refuse to lightly trim or dust the ends of your hair while your ends are splitting or breaking, in no time you will have stringy thin hair and this will cause you to lose more length that could have been preserved!

When it comes to the Big Chop, this can be a very freeing process for many who are transitioning. In most cases, long term transitioning and trimming off hair gradually overtime, will eventually help you reach your goal of 100% natural hair. A Big Chop just gets you to fully natural hair faster!

Big chopping is suggested for those who don't have much patience in regards to maintaining their hair because maintaining one texture of hair is a lot easier than managing two. Also big chopping is suggested for those who have chronically damaged relaxed hair or for those who want to have natural hair as fast as possible.

I will walk you step by step through Big Chopping and give you some tips and direction on how to successfully do so without cutting off unnecessary hair!

ONLY USE CUTTING SHEARS EXCLUSIVELY ON YOUR TRANSITIONING HAIR!

Step #1 Begin with freshly washed damp product free hair. The line of demarcation is most prevalent if you hair has is product free and has not been stretched or styled.

Step #2 Starting on one side of your head and working your way towards the other side, begin clipping away relaxed hair in small sections without pulling your hair whatsoever. Just to make sure the very ends of your hair are not still relaxed, slightly pull your section of hair and clip barely above your line of demarcation.

Step #3 After trimming, detangle small sections of hair at a time while damp with your seamless wide tooth detangling comb to check for straight ends that were left behind. Trim as needed.

Step #4 If you feel comfortable having someone else give you a Big Chop, have a friend or professional assist you with your transformation!

AFTERWORDS

"This manual was made in mind for those who desire step by step help with Transitioning from Relaxed Hair to Natural Hair! You may have chosen to read this guide because you support my work, you were looking for information on Transitioning, or you were looking for this information to help a loved one. Personally, I transitioned from relaxed to natural hair without even realizing it! At the time when I was transitioning, I did not know that I was doing that very thing. I decided around 17 or 18 years old to stop chemically relaxing my hair because I was tired of the pain and constant breakage I was experiencing from relaxers. There were times when I was able to manage the effects the chemicals had on my hair and scalp, but it progressively became intolerable due to the fact that I had mild scalp eczema.

At the beginning stages of growing my natural hair, I wished I had a book like this that could point me in the direction that could help me better care for my hair! I did not grow up around women with natural hair so many lessons were learned from my experience. Even though I had a lack of information earlier on in my life, I decided to seek education about hair and learn how to keep it healthy in a variety of ways hair could possibly be worn! In my book, The Natural Hair Bible and The Relaxed Hair Bible, I discuss in great depth, and detail about the fundamentals of hair care beyond the scope of this easy to read manual if you desire more information on hair care and hairstyling.

I hope that you thoroughly enjoyed this read, it was a pleasure of mine to write this for your knowledge and enjoyment."

Sincerely, Breanna

ADDITIONAL RESOURCES

The Official Website: www.Howtoblackhair.com

The Online Store: www.HowtoblackhairStore.com

Free Subscription Email: http://eepurl.com/FZs5b

For Additional Hair Questions

YourHairQuestions@Gmail.com

Black Hair Styling Tutorials

BlackWomenHair YouTube Channel

www.Youtube.com/BlackWomenHair

HowToBlackHair YouTube Channel

www.Youtube.com/HowToBlackHair

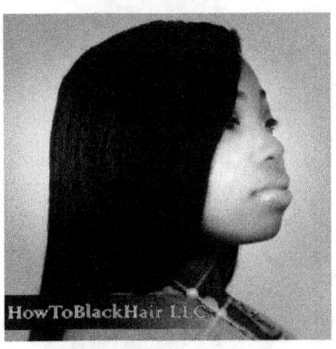

The Natural Hair Bible

The 10 Commandments of Black Hair Care

www.HowToBlackHair.com

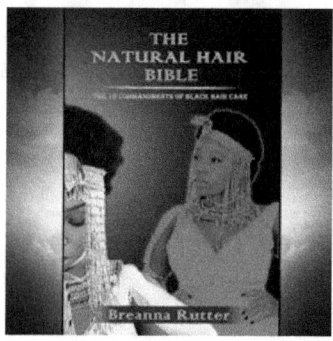

The Relaxed Hair Bible

The 10 Commandments of Long Healthy Relaxed Hair

www.HowToBlackHair.com

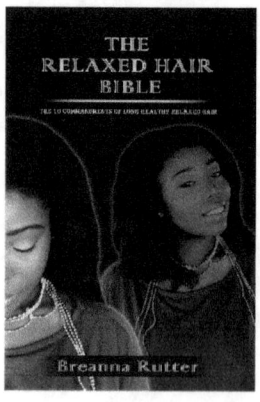

Black Hair Styling DVDs (Over 20+ Hairstyles)

www.HowToBlackHair.com

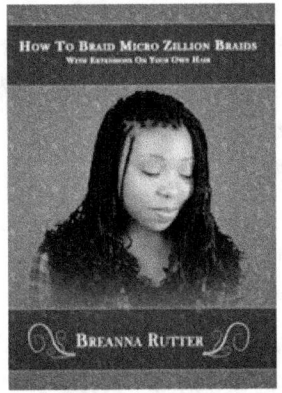 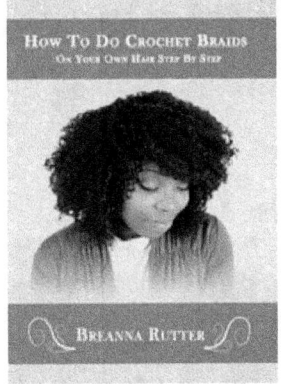

DEFINITION GUIDE

Big Chop: *cutting off all of your relaxed hair while your natural hair remains*

Buildup: *hair care products, sweat, dirt, oils, and/or skin that has gathered on your hair and scalp*

Chase Method: *a method of straightening hair with one pass of the flat iron by following the flat iron closely behind the drag of a rat tail comb*

Color Treated: *hair that has been colored*

Curl Pattern: *the natural curl pattern of your hair strands according to the LOIS or Andre Walker hair typing system*

Cuticles: *a naturally protecting shield (arranged like shingles to the roof of a home) outside of your hair strands*

Dry Detangle: *detangling without moisture or with just oils*

Dusting: *trimming about an 1/8 inch of hair from the ends*

Elasticity: *the stretching ability of your hair*

Fine Hair: *your individual strands of hair are closer in size (circumference) to string instead of thread*

Hair Shaft: *the visibly seen strands of hair*

Hair Type: *identifying your hair based on the texture (feel) and curl pattern (look)*

Heat Damage: *using heat that causes hair to no longer revert to your original curl pattern*

Heat Trained: *using heat overtime on hair to make hair permanently straight*

Loc Method: *layering products for moisture in the order of; Liquid (leave in moisturizer or water), Oil, Cream (thick consistency moisturizer/sealant like a hair butter).*

Line of Demarcation: *the meeting point of division between relaxed hair and natural hair or color treated hair and natural hair color*

Natural Hair: *hair that is not treated with a chemical relaxer*

New Growth: *distinguishable unrelaxed hair growth whether relaxed or natural*

Regimen: *a collection of hair care tools, products, and practices that contribute to hair growth*

Relaxed Hair: *hair that is treated with a relaxer*
Retain Length: *using a regimen that allows hair to grow faster than the rate of breakage or trimming*
Retain Moisture: *the ability to prevent hair from becoming dry*
Revert: *hair that returns back to its curl pattern*
Roots: *new growth*
Shrinkage: *hair shrinking in contact of moisture*
Tension Method: *holding hair stretched with your hand when blow drying*
Transitioning: *going natural while trimming relaxed ends to your level of comfort without the big chop*
Type 3 Hair: *hair that looks like curls instead of a coils*
Type 4 Hair: *hair that looks like coils or kinks instead of curls*

INDEX

HOW TO BLACK HAIR LLC.
WRITTEN BY BREANNA RUTTER
BOOK DESIGNED BY BREANNA RUTTER
COVER DESIGNED BY JARED RUTTER
ALL RIGHTS RESERVED.
VISIT WWW.HOWTOBLACKHAIR.COM

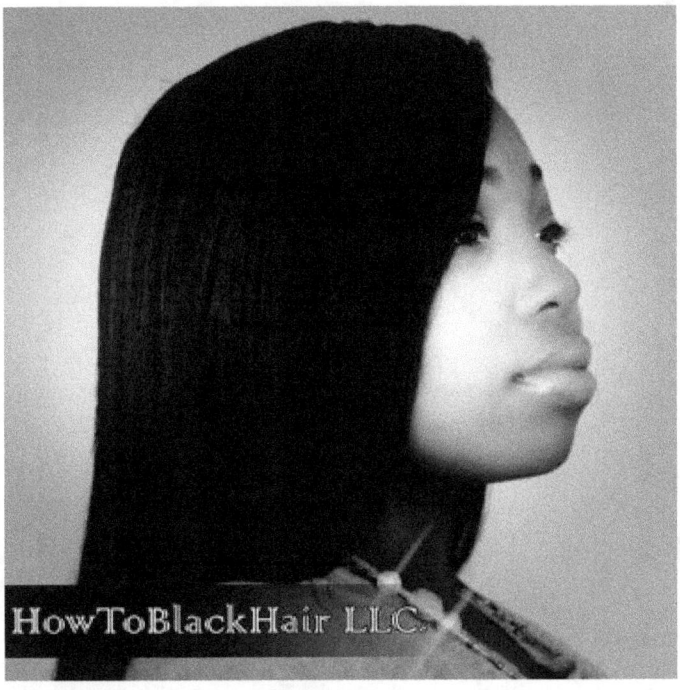